T0145307

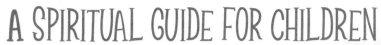

A SPIRITUAL GUIDE FOR CHILDREN

FEEL YOUR WAY THROUGH LIFE

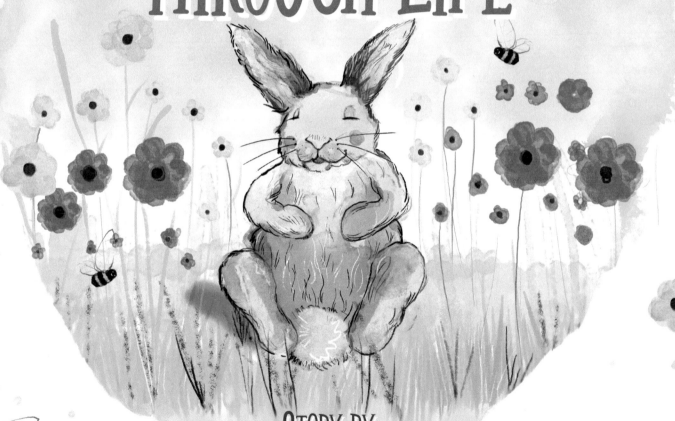

STORY BY
ANNEKARIEN VAN DE VELDE

ILLUSTRATIONS BY ELENA PĂUN

Balboa Press books may be ordered through booksellers or by contacting:

Balboa Press
A Division of Hay House
1663 Liberty Drive
Bloomington, IN 47403
www.balboapress.com
1 (877) 407–4847

ISBN: 978-1-5043-1422-0 (sc)
ISBN: 978-1-5043-1423-7 (e)

Print information available on the last page.

Balboa Press rev. date: 08/17/2018

BALBOA
PRESS
A DIVISION OF HAY HOUSE

For Viggo, Lars and Julia
who I love dearly

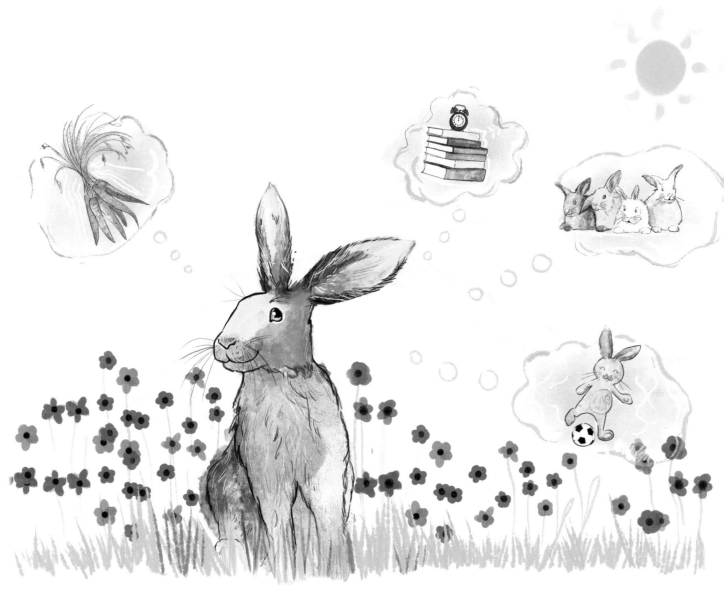

When my head gets busy with thoughts, I stop.

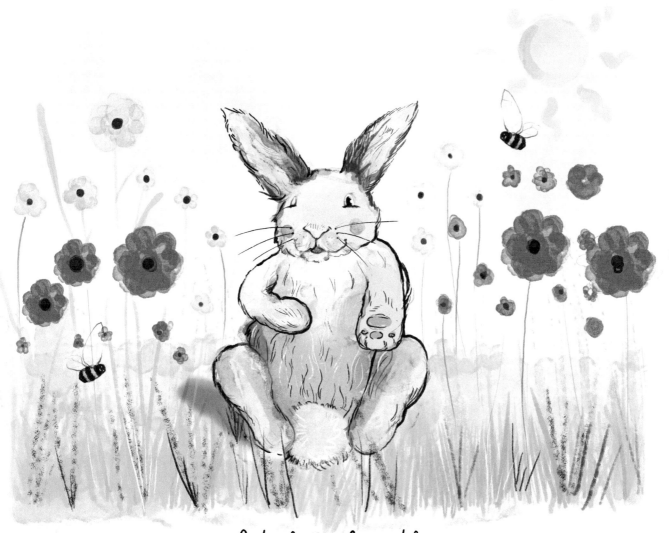

I take a breath.
Will you join me?

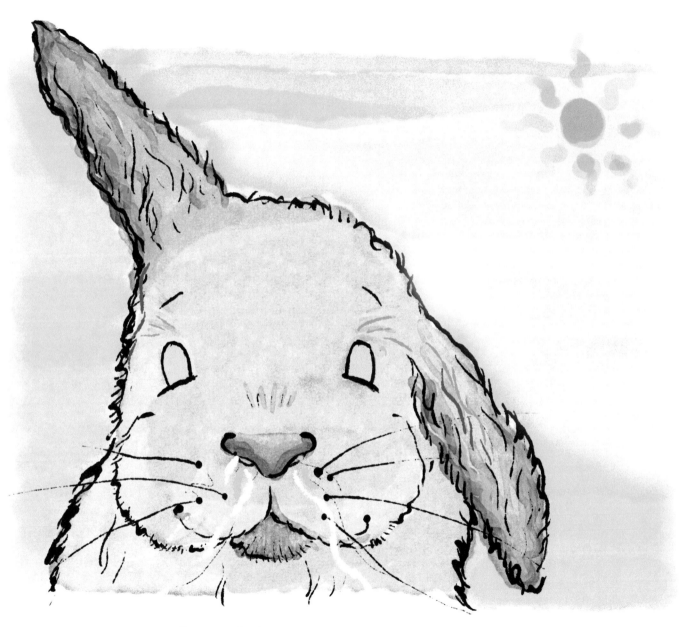

I feel the air going up my nose.
Can you feel that too?

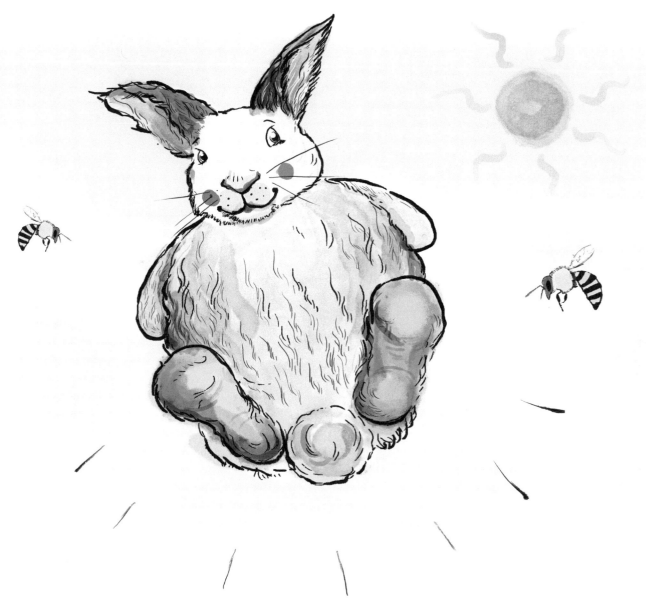

My chest and my belly rise as they fill up with air.
It is as if a balloon is being blown up inside me.

I feel the flow of air stop briefly...
And then I feel the air flow out of my mouth.
My chest and belly go flat.
Did you notice that too?

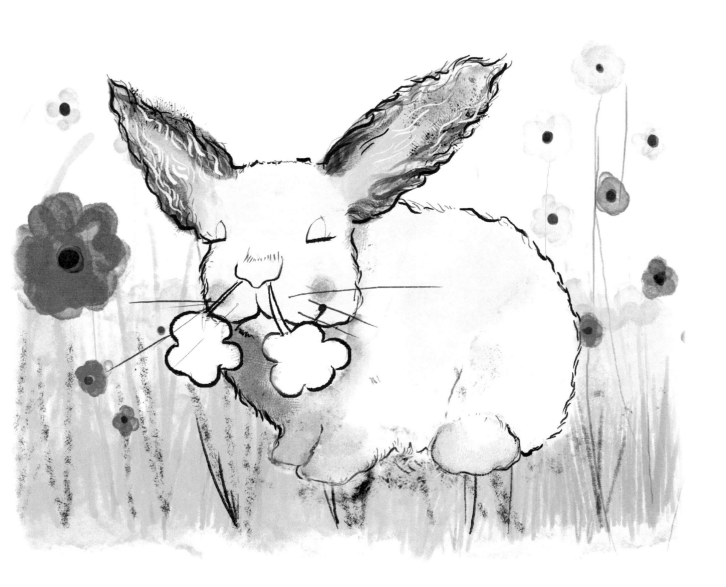

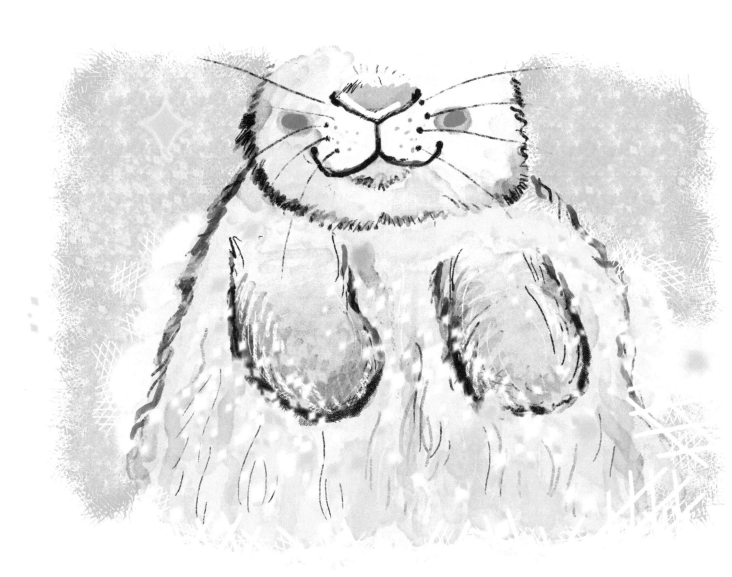

I focus on my hands.
I feel the energy in my hands.

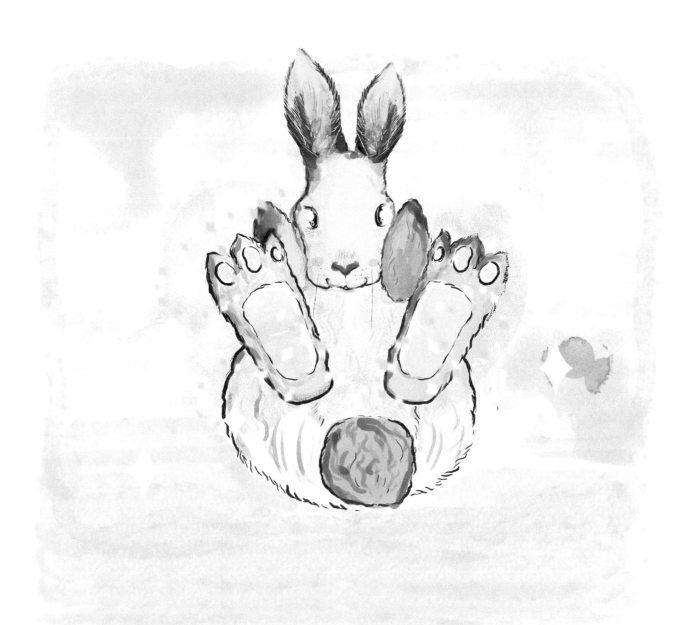

I focus on my feet.
I feel the energy in my feet.
Can you feel this too?

My mind gets busy sometimes.
Then I think about many things.
And that is totally normal and perfectly fine.

But I am not my mind. I am not my thoughts.
And you are not your mind. You
are not your thoughts.

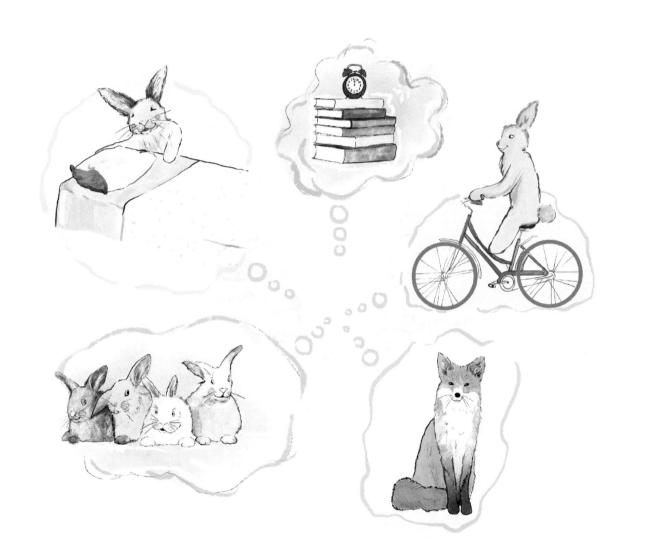

My mind and my thoughts
are like a television.
But I am not a television.

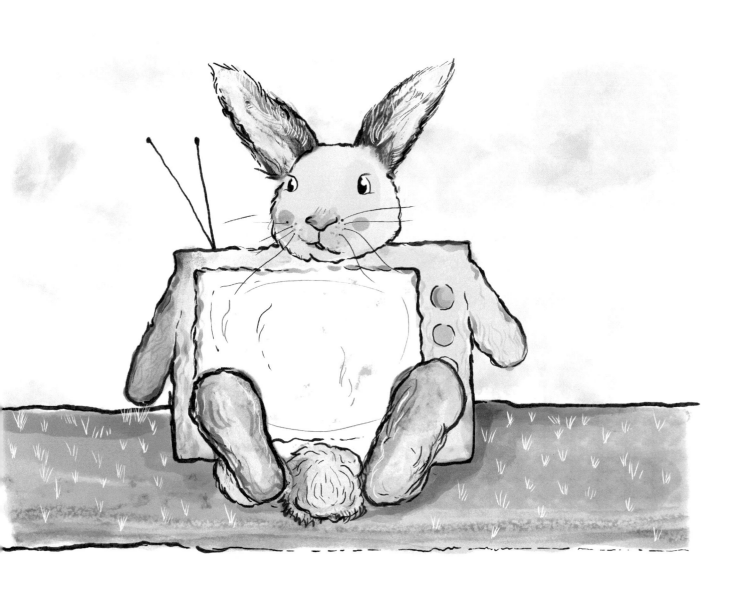

The real me is watching the television.

You are not a television either, are you?
The real you is watching the television too.

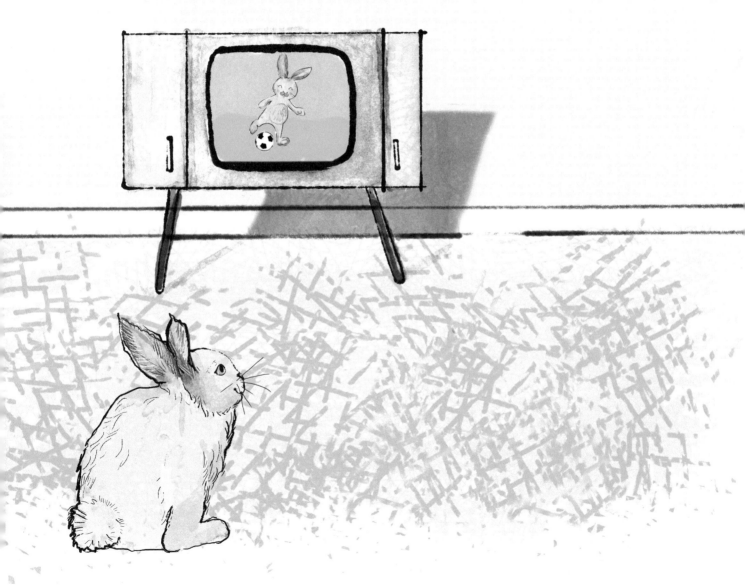

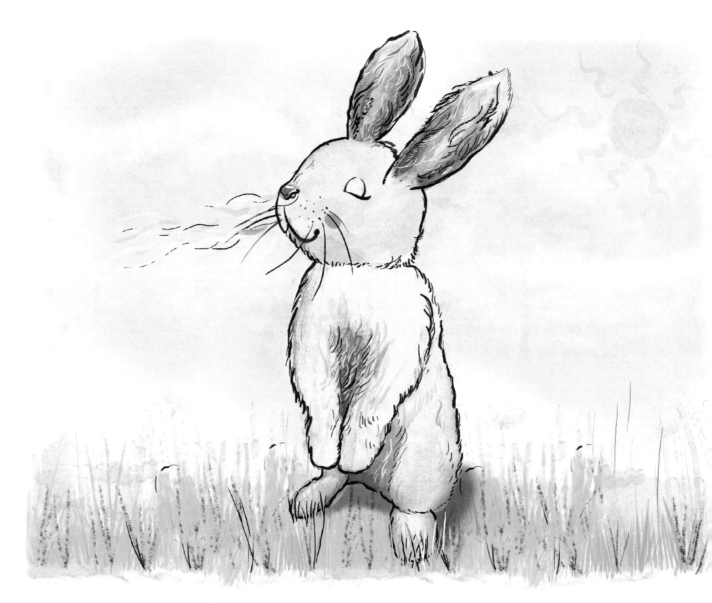

When I focus on my breath,
I feel the real me.

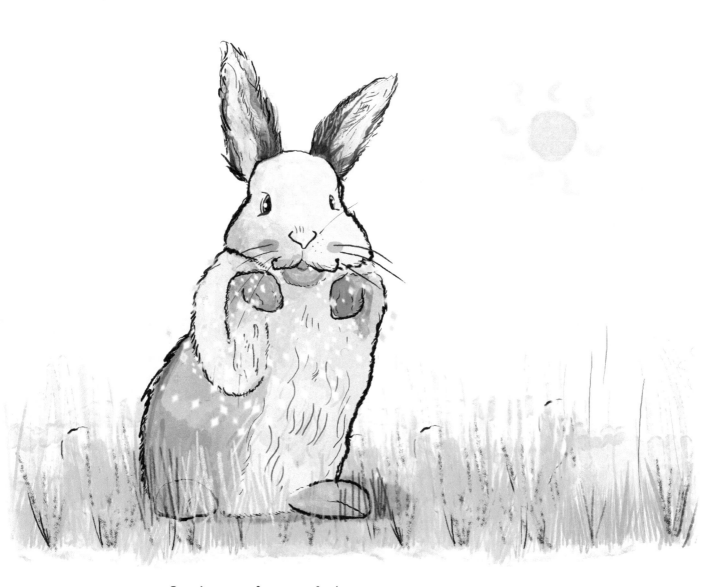

When I feel the energy in my
hands, I feel the real me.

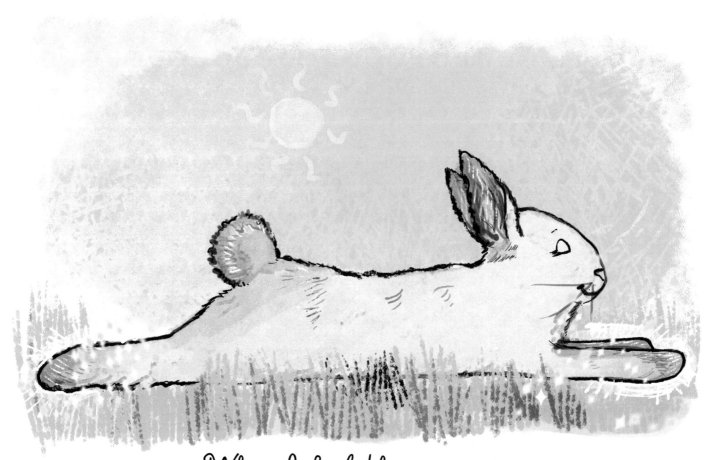

When I feel the energy in my
feet, I feel the real me.

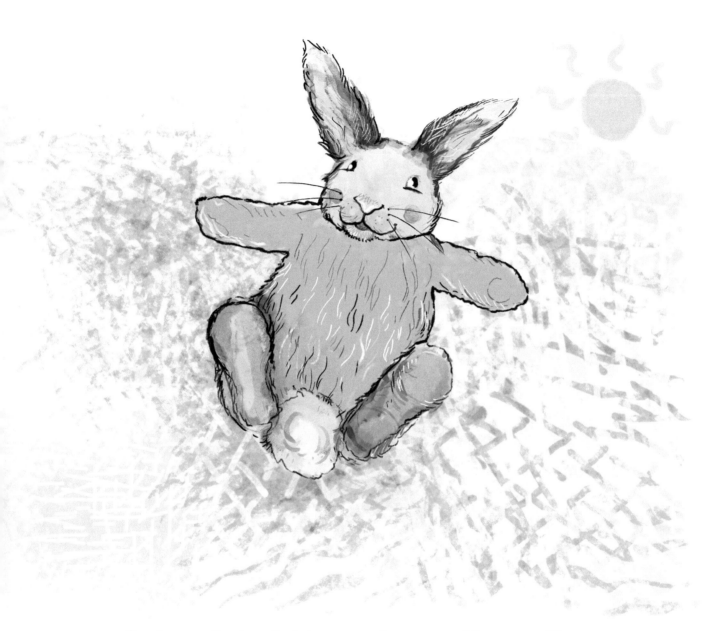

When I feel the real me, all is well.

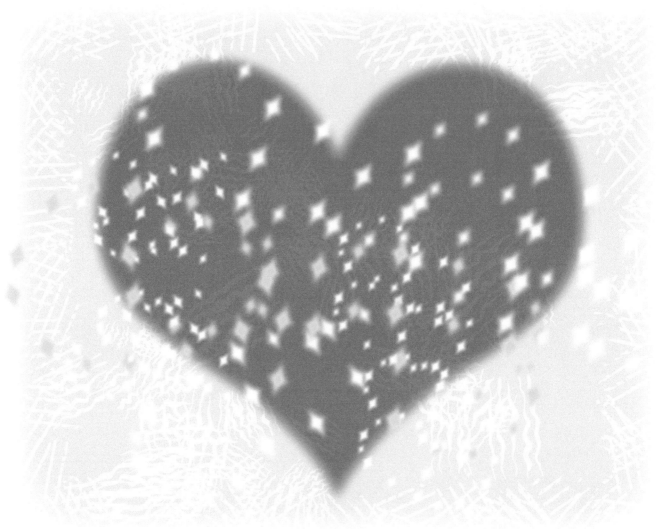

And when you feel the real you, all is well.
Yes...

All is well!

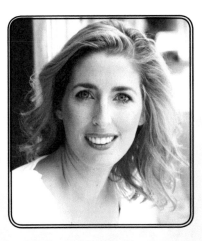

Annekarien is passionate about bringing a simplified form of spiritual wisdom to children, so it can be part of their life's journey from an early age. Annekarien was born in The Netherlands and currently resides in New Zealand with her husband and their three children.

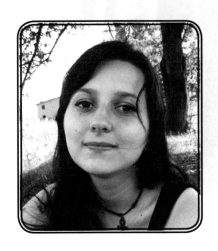

Elena is an Illustrator, graphic designer and artist. She is based in Iasi, Romania.

Printed in the United States
By Bookmasters